MENOPAUSE DIET COOKBOOK

Dr. Kimberly Carlos

Copyright © 2023 by Dr. Kimberly Carlos

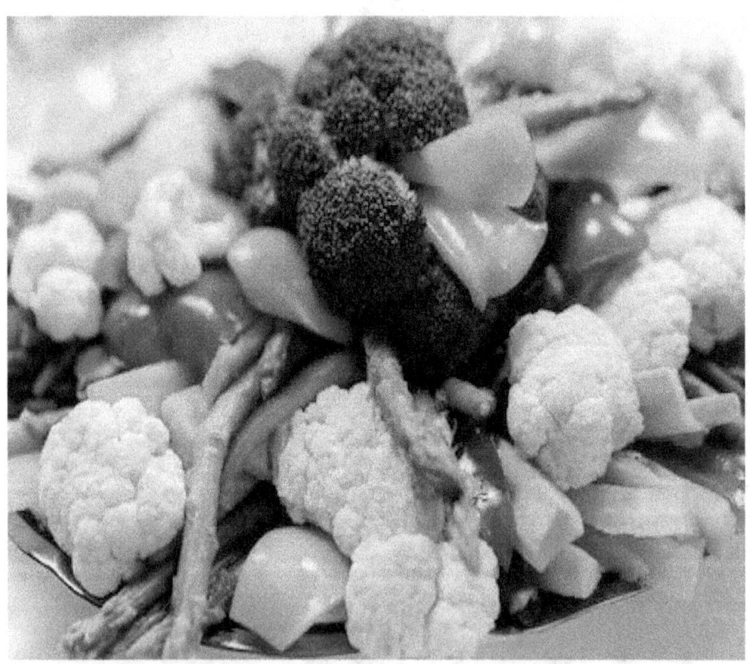

TABLE OF CONTENT

INTRODUCTION

Sarah had always been an active and vibrant woman, but as she approached her 50s, the onset of menopause brought about a wave of changes she hadn't anticipated. Hot flashes, mood swings, and weight gain seemed to be taking over her life. Determined to regain control and embrace this new phase, Sarah decided to explore the power of a menopause diet.

She started by researching foods that could alleviate her symptoms. Fresh fruits and vegetables became her daily companions, offering a rich source of vitamins and minerals. Leafy greens, berries, and citrus fruits quickly became staples in her diet, helping her combat the fatigue that often accompanied menopause.

Protein-rich foods like lean meats, fish, and legumes became crucial for maintaining her muscle mass and energy levels. Sarah also added more calcium and vitamin D to her diet, which helped improve her bone health and reduce the risk of osteoporosis.

To manage her hot flashes and mood swings, Sarah included foods rich in phytoestrogens, such as soy products and flaxseeds. These natural compounds mimicked estrogen's effects, balancing her hormones and reducing the intensity of her symptoms.

Incorporating healthy fats like avocados and nuts into her diet not only supported her heart health but also helped control her weight. With portion control and mindful eating, Sarah watched as the extra pounds she'd gained during menopause began to melt away.

As the weeks turned into months, Sarah felt like a new person. Her hot flashes had become less frequent, and her mood swings were far more manageable. Her renewed energy and zest for life were infectious, inspiring her friends to explore the benefits of a menopause diet as well.

Through a simple change in her eating habits, Sarah had not only embraced menopause but also found a healthier, happier version of herself. The menopause diet had become her secret weapon in navigating this new chapter of her life with grace and vitality.

CHAPTER ONE

Following a Menopause Diet with Benefits

Following a menopause diet with benefits involves making mindful dietary choices to manage the symptoms and health challenges associated with menopause.

Here are some tips on how to do that:

1. Consult a Healthcare Professional: Before making any significant dietary changes, consult with a healthcare provider or a registered dietitian who can assess your specific needs, health status, and dietary preferences. They can help you create a personalized menopause diet plan.

2. Balanced Nutrition: Focus on a well-balanced diet that includes a variety of foods from all food groups. This should include:

- Fruits and Vegetables: Incorporate plenty of fruits and vegetables into your daily meals for essential vitamins, minerals, and fiber.
- Lean Proteins: Choose lean sources of protein like poultry, fish, beans, and tofu to support muscle mass and overall health.

- Whole Grains: Opt for whole grains such as brown rice, whole wheat, and oats to provide sustained energy and fiber.
- Healthy Fats: Include sources of healthy fats like avocados, nuts, seeds, and olive oil to support heart health.
- Dairy or Dairy Alternatives: Ensure you get enough calcium and vitamin D through dairy products or fortified dairy alternatives to support bone health.

3. Phytoestrogen-Rich Foods: Incorporate foods rich in phytoestrogens, like soy products, flaxseeds, and legumes. These can help balance hormone levels and reduce menopausal symptoms.

4. Hydration: Stay hydrated by drinking plenty of water throughout the day. Limit caffeine and alcohol intake, as these can exacerbate hot flashes and affect sleep.

5. Portion Control: Be mindful of portion sizes to manage your weight, as metabolism tends to slow down during menopause. Smaller, balanced meals can help prevent weight gain.

6. Limit Processed Foods: Minimize your consumption of processed and sugary foods, as they can contribute to weight gain and exacerbate mood swings.

7. Regular Exercise: Combine your menopause diet with regular physical activity. Exercise can help maintain muscle mass, reduce stress, and boost your mood.

8. Bone Health: Pay special attention to calcium and vitamin D intake, as bone density tends to decrease during menopause. Dairy products, leafy greens, and fortified foods can help.

9. Mindful Eating: Practice mindful eating by paying attention to hunger and fullness cues. This can prevent overeating and promote better digestion.

10. Supplements: Talk to your healthcare provider about the need for supplements, such as calcium, vitamin D, or omega-3 fatty acids, based on your individual requirements.

11. Track Your Progress: Keep a journal to monitor your symptoms, diet, and how you feel. This can help you identify which dietary changes are most effective for your specific needs.

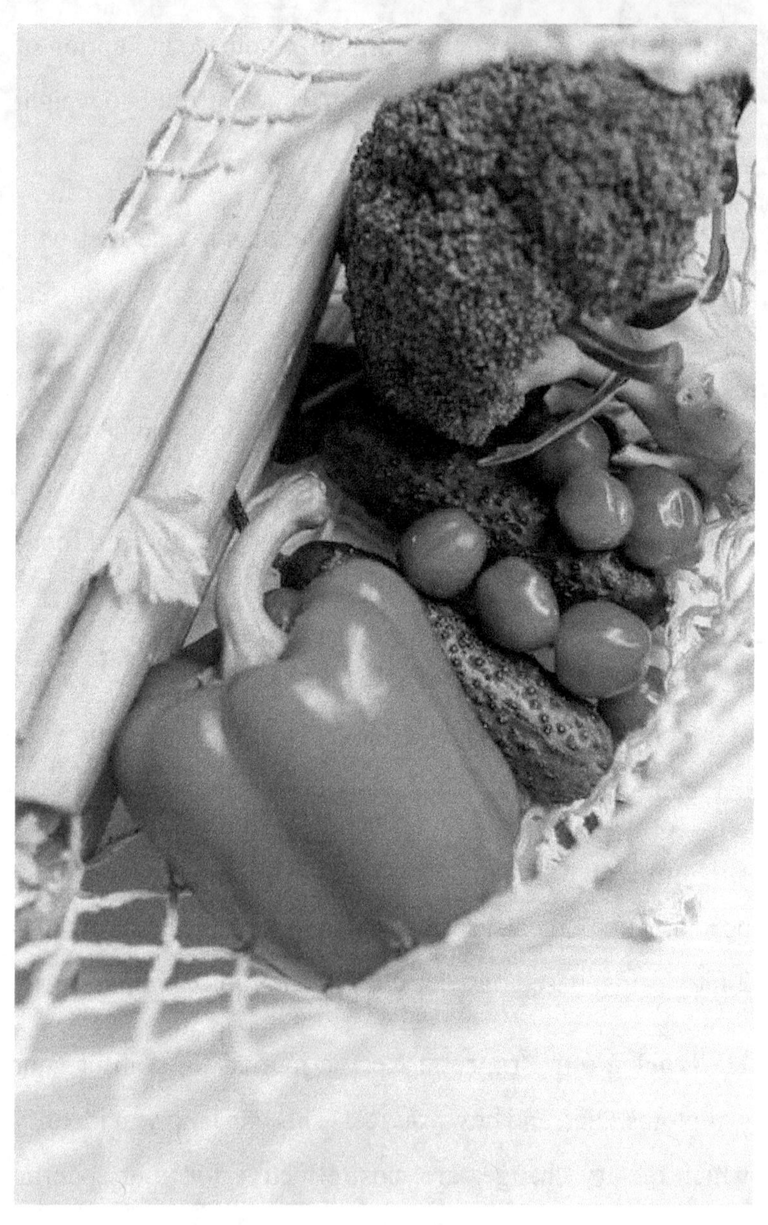

CHAPTER TWO

14-Day Menopause Diet Meal Plan

Day 1:

- Breakfast: Greek yogurt with berries and a sprinkle of flaxseeds.
- Lunch: Spinach and quinoa salad with grilled chicken and balsamic vinaigrette.
- Snack: Carrot and cucumber sticks with hummus.
- Dinner: Baked salmon with steamed broccoli and brown rice.

Day 2:

- Breakfast: Oatmeal topped with sliced bananas and almonds.
- Lunch: Lentil soup and a mixed greens salad with chickpeas.
- Snack: Greek yogurt with honey.
- Dinner: Stir-fried tofu with mixed vegetables and quinoa.

Day 3:

- Breakfast: Scrambled eggs with spinach and whole-grain toast.

- Lunch: Turkey and avocado wrap with a side of vegetable sticks.

- Snack: Mixed nuts (portion-controlled).

- Dinner: Grilled shrimp with asparagus and a quinoa pilaf.

Day 4:

- Breakfast: Smoothie with spinach, frozen berries, Greek yogurt, and a scoop of protein powder.

- Lunch: Quinoa and black bean salad with a lime-cilantro dressing.

- Snack: Sliced pear with a sprinkle of cinnamon.

- Dinner: Baked chicken breast with roasted sweet potatoes and green beans.

Day 5:

- Breakfast: Cottage cheese with sliced peaches and a drizzle of honey.

- Lunch: Spinach and feta stuffed chicken breast with a side of steamed broccoli.

- Snack: Edamame (portion-controlled).

- Dinner: Baked cod with quinoa and sautéed spinach.

Day 6:

- Breakfast: Whole-grain cereal with almond milk and fresh strawberries.
- Lunch: Tuna salad with mixed greens and whole-grain crackers.
- Snack: Sliced cucumber with tzatziki sauce.
- Dinner: Grilled steak with roasted Brussels sprouts and a quinoa pilaf.

Day 7:

- Breakfast: Scrambled eggs with diced tomatoes and avocado.
- Lunch: Chickpea and vegetable curry with brown rice.
- Snack: Mixed berries with a dollop of Greek yogurt.
- Dinner: Baked tilapia with asparagus and a side of couscous.

Day 8:

- Breakfast: Greek yogurt with sliced peaches and a drizzle of honey.
- Lunch: Quinoa and roasted vegetable bowl with a tahini dressing.

- Snack: Baby carrots and cherry tomatoes with a light ranch dip.
- Dinner: Grilled chicken breast with a side of sautéed kale and brown rice.

Day 9:

- Breakfast: Smoothie with kale, banana, almond milk, and chia seeds.
- Lunch: Spinach and mushroom whole-grain pasta with a tomato sauce.
- Snack: Sliced apple with a tablespoon of almond butter.
- Dinner: Baked cod with a lemon herb crust, served with quinoa and steamed asparagus.

Day 10:

- Breakfast: Scrambled eggs with diced bell peppers and a whole-grain English muffin.
- Lunch: Turkey and avocado salad with mixed greens and a light vinaigrette.
- Snack: Mixed nuts and dried cranberries (portion-controlled).
- Dinner: Grilled shrimp with a quinoa and vegetable

stir-fry.

Day 11:

- Breakfast: Overnight oats made with oats, almond milk, chia seeds, and topped with sliced strawberries.
- Lunch: Lentil and vegetable stew with a side of whole-grain bread.
- Snack: Sliced cucumber and red pepper with hummus.
- Dinner: Baked chicken thighs with roasted Brussels sprouts and quinoa.

Day 12:

- Breakfast: Cottage cheese with pineapple chunks and a sprinkle of cinnamon.
- Lunch: Spinach and feta stuffed turkey burger on a whole-grain bun with a side salad.
- Snack: A small bowl of mixed berries.
- Dinner: Baked salmon with a dill yogurt sauce, served with quinoa and steamed broccoli.

Day 13:

- Breakfast: Smoothie with spinach, banana, almond

milk, and a scoop of protein powder.

- Lunch: Chickpea and kale salad with lemon-tahini dressing.
- Snack: Sliced pear with a slice of low-fat cheese.
- Dinner: Grilled steak with a mixed vegetable stir-fry and brown rice.

Day 14:

- Breakfast: Scrambled eggs with diced tomatoes and a slice of whole-grain toast.
- Lunch: Tuna and white bean salad with mixed greens and a balsamic vinaigrette.
- Snack: A small handful of almonds (portion-controlled).
- Dinner: Baked tilapia with quinoa and sautéed spinach.

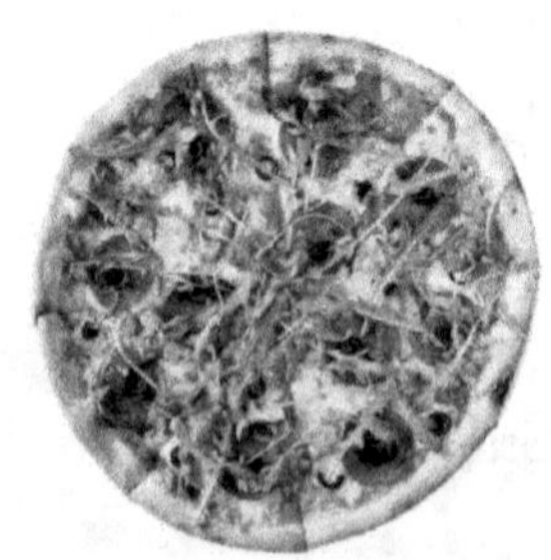

CHAPTER THREE

Menopause diet Breakfast Recipes

1. Berry Breakfast Parfait

A delightful and nutritious way to start your day during menopause, this parfait is packed with antioxidants and fiber to help manage symptoms.

Ingredients:

- 1 cup Greek yogurt
- 1/2 cup mixed berries (strawberries, blueberries, raspberries)
- 1/4 cup granola
- 1 tablespoon honey

Instructions:

1. In a glass or bowl, layer Greek yogurt.

2. Add a layer of mixed berries on top of the yogurt.

3. Sprinkle granola over the berries.

4. Drizzle honey over the top.

5. Serve immediately.

Cooking Time: 5 minutes

2. Spinach and Mushroom Omelette

Packed with iron and protein, this omelette provides the energy and nutrients needed to tackle the day's challenges.

Ingredients:

- 2 large eggs
- 1/2 cup fresh spinach, chopped
- 1/4 cup sliced mushrooms
- 2 tablespoons diced red bell pepper
- Salt and pepper to taste
- Cooking spray

Instructions:

1. In a bowl, whisk eggs and season with salt and pepper.

2. Heat a non-stick skillet over medium heat and lightly coat with cooking spray.

3. Add mushrooms and red bell pepper, sauté until tender.

4. Pour the whisked eggs over the veggies.

5. Sprinkle chopped spinach over one half of the omelette.

6. Cook until the eggs are set, then fold the omelette in half.

7. Serve hot.

Cooking Time: 10 minutes

3. Chia Seed Pudding

Chia seeds are rich in omega-3 fatty acids and fiber, making this pudding a satisfying and heart-healthy breakfast option.

Ingredients:

- 2 tablespoons chia seeds
- 1 cup almond milk (or any milk of your choice)
- 1/2 teaspoon vanilla extract
- 1 tablespoon honey
- Fresh fruit for topping (e.g., sliced strawberries, kiwi)

Instructions:

1. In a bowl, combine chia seeds, almond milk, vanilla extract, and honey.

2. Stir well, then cover and refrigerate overnight.

3. In the morning, give it a good stir and top with fresh fruit.

Cooking Time: 5 minutes (plus overnight refrigeration)

4. Quinoa Breakfast Bowl

Quinoa is a great source of protein and fiber, and this bowl is a fantastic way to start your day with sustained energy.

Ingredients:

- 1/2 cup cooked quinoa
- 1/4 cup Greek yogurt
- 1/4 cup sliced bananas
- 1 tablespoon chopped nuts (e.g., almonds or walnuts)
- 1 tablespoon honey or maple syrup

Instructions:

1. In a bowl, layer cooked quinoa.

2. Top with Greek yogurt.

3. Add sliced bananas and chopped nuts.

4. Drizzle with honey or maple syrup.

5. Enjoy!

Cooking Time: 15 minutes (if quinoa is not pre-cooked)

5. Overnight Oats

A quick and convenient breakfast option, these oats are loaded with fiber and nutrients to keep you feeling full and satisfied.

Ingredients:

- 1/2 cup rolled oats
- 1/2 cup almond milk (or any milk of your choice)
- 1/2 cup diced apples
- 1 tablespoon chia seeds
- 1/2 teaspoon cinnamon
- 1 tablespoon honey or agave nectar

Instructions:

1. In a jar or bowl, combine rolled oats, almond milk, diced apples, chia seeds, and cinnamon.

2. Stir well, then cover and refrigerate overnight.

3. In the morning, drizzle with honey or agave nectar before serving.

Cooking Time: 5 minutes (plus overnight refrigeration)

6. Veggie Breakfast Burrito

This savory breakfast burrito is rich in fiber and protein, helping you stay full and focused throughout the morning.

Ingredients:

- 1 whole wheat tortilla
- 2 large eggs
- 1/4 cup diced bell peppers
- 1/4 cup diced onions
- 1/4 cup black beans (canned, drained, and rinsed)
- 2 tablespoons salsa
- Salt and pepper to taste
- Cooking spray

Instructions:

1. In a skillet, heat cooking spray over medium heat.

2. Add diced bell peppers and onions, sauté until tender.

3. In a bowl, whisk eggs and add to the skillet.

4. Scramble eggs, then add black beans and salsa.

5. Season with salt and pepper.

6. Spoon the egg and veggie mixture onto the tortilla, fold, and serve.

Cooking Time: 15 minutes

7. Avocado Toast with Poached Egg

Avocado is a great source of healthy fats, and when paired with a poached egg, it creates a balanced and satisfying breakfast.

Ingredients:

- 1 slice whole-grain bread
- 1/2 ripe avocado, mashed
- 1 poached egg
- Salt and pepper to taste
- Optional toppings: crushed red pepper flakes, sliced tomatoes

Instructions:

1. Toast the whole-grain bread.

2. Spread the mashed avocado on the toast.

3. Top with a poached egg.

4. Season with salt and pepper.

5. Add optional toppings if desired.

6. Serve immediately.

Cooking Time: 10 minutes (including poaching the egg)

8. Banana Walnut Pancakes

These whole-grain pancakes are a comforting breakfast choice and provide potassium and healthy fats.

Ingredients:

- 1/2 cup whole-wheat pancake mix
- 1/2 ripe banana, mashed
- 1/4 cup chopped walnuts
- 1/2 cup almond milk (or any milk of your choice)
- Cooking spray

Instructions:

1. In a bowl, combine pancake mix, mashed banana, chopped walnuts, and almond milk.

2. Mix until just combined.

3. Heat a griddle or non-stick skillet over medium heat, lightly coated with cooking spray.

4. Pour pancake batter onto the griddle to make small pancakes.

5. Cook until bubbles form on the surface, then flip and cook until golden brown.

6. Serve with a drizzle of honey or maple syrup if desired.

Cooking Time: 15 minutes

9. Smoked Salmon and Cream Cheese Bagel

This classic breakfast offers a dose of omega-3 fatty acids and protein, perfect for a special morning treat.

Ingredients:

- 1 whole wheat bagel
- 2 tablespoons low-fat cream cheese
- 2 slices smoked salmon
- Sliced cucumber and red onion (optional)
- Fresh dill for garnish (optional)

Instructions:

1. Toast the whole wheat bagel.

2. Spread cream cheese on both bagel halves.

3. Layer smoked salmon on one half.

4. Add optional cucumber and red onion slices.

5. Garnish with fresh dill if desired.

6. Assemble the bagel, slice, and serve.

Cooking Time: 5 minutes

10. Blueberry Almond Breakfast Quinoa

Quinoa isn't just for savory dishes; it's a fantastic base for a sweet, satisfying breakfast loaded with antioxidants and protein.

Ingredients:

- 1/2 cup cooked quinoa
- 1/4 cup almond milk (or any milk of your choice)
- 1/4 cup fresh blueberries
- 1 tablespoon sliced almonds

- 1/2 teaspoon honey or maple syrup

- 1/4 teaspoon vanilla extract

Instructions:

1. In a bowl, combine cooked quinoa, almond milk, fresh blueberries, sliced almonds, honey or maple syrup, and vanilla extract.

2. Stir well.

3. Microwave for 1-2 minutes until warm.

4. Serve as a nutritious breakfast bowl.

Cooking Time: 5 minutes

Menopause Diet Lunch Recipes

1. Quinoa and Black Bean Salad

A protein-packed salad that's rich in fiber and essential nutrients to keep you energized during the day.

Ingredients:

- 1 cup cooked quinoa

- 1 can (15 oz) black beans, drained and rinsed

- 1 cup corn kernels (fresh or frozen)

- 1 red bell pepper, diced
- 1/2 cup cherry tomatoes, halved
- 1/4 cup fresh cilantro, chopped
- Juice of 1 lime
- 2 tablespoons olive oil
- Salt and pepper to taste

Instructions:

1. In a large bowl, combine cooked quinoa, black beans, corn, red bell pepper, cherry tomatoes, and cilantro.

2. In a small bowl, whisk together lime juice, olive oil, salt, and pepper to create the dressing.

3. Drizzle the dressing over the salad and toss gently to combine.

4. Serve chilled.

Cooking Time: 20 minutes (if quinoa is not pre-cooked)

2. Salmon and Asparagus Foil Packets

A simple and healthy lunch option that's rich in omega-3 fatty acids and essential vitamins.

Ingredients:

- 2 salmon fillets
- 1 bunch asparagus, trimmed
- 1 lemon, thinly sliced
- 2 cloves garlic, minced
- Fresh dill or parsley for garnish
- Salt and pepper to taste
- Olive oil for drizzling

Instructions:

1. Preheat the oven to 375°F (190°C).

2. Place each salmon fillet on a separate sheet of aluminum foil.

3. Season the salmon with minced garlic, salt, and pepper.

4. Arrange asparagus spears and lemon slices around each salmon fillet.

5. Drizzle with olive oil.

6. Fold the foil to create packets, sealing them tightly.

7. Bake for 15-20 minutes or until salmon is cooked through.

8. Garnish with fresh dill or parsley before serving.

Cooking Time: 20-25 minutes

3. Spinach and Feta Stuffed Chicken Breast

A flavorful and protein-packed lunch option to support your muscle health during menopause.

Ingredients:

- 2 boneless, skinless chicken breasts
- 1 cup fresh spinach leaves
- 1/4 cup crumbled feta cheese
- 1 teaspoon olive oil
- 1/2 teaspoon garlic powder
- 1/2 teaspoon dried oregano
- Salt and pepper to taste

Instructions:

1. Preheat the oven to 375°F (190°C).

2. Cut a pocket into each chicken breast.

3. Stuff each pocket with fresh spinach and feta cheese.

4. Rub the outside of the chicken breasts with olive oil, garlic powder, dried oregano, salt, and pepper.

5. Place the stuffed chicken breasts in a baking dish.

6. Bake for 25-30 minutes or until the chicken is cooked through and no longer pink.

7. Serve hot.

Cooking Time: 30-35 minutes

4. Lentil and Vegetable Stir-Fry

A plant-based lunch option that's rich in fiber, protein, and essential nutrients.

Ingredients:

- 1 cup cooked green or brown lentils
- 2 cups mixed vegetables (e.g., bell peppers, broccoli, carrots)
- 2 cloves garlic, minced
- 1 tablespoon ginger, minced
- 2 tablespoons low-sodium soy sauce or tamari
- 1 tablespoon sesame oil
- 1 teaspoon honey or agave nectar
- Sesame seeds for garnish
- Cooked brown rice or quinoa (optional)

Instructions:

1. Heat sesame oil in a large skillet or wok over medium-high heat.

2. Add minced garlic and ginger; stir-fry for 30 seconds.

3. Add mixed vegetables and stir-fry for 3-4 minutes or until tender-crisp.

4. In a small bowl, whisk together soy sauce and honey or agave nectar.

5. Add the cooked lentils to the skillet, pour the sauce over the lentils and vegetables, and stir well.

6. Cook for an additional 2-3 minutes to heat through.

7. Serve as is or over cooked brown rice or quinoa.

8. Garnish with sesame seeds.

Cooking Time: 20 minutes (if lentils are not pre-cooked)

5. Tuna and White Bean Salad

A protein-packed salad that's easy to prepare and perfect for a quick and nutritious lunch.

Ingredients:

- 2 cans (5 oz each) tuna, drained

- 1 can (15 oz) white beans (cannellini or Great Northern), drained and rinsed
- 1/2 red onion, finely chopped
- 1/4 cup fresh parsley, chopped
- Juice of 1 lemon
- 2 tablespoons olive oil
- Salt and pepper to taste
- Mixed greens for serving

Instructions:

1. In a large bowl, combine tuna, white beans, red onion, and parsley.

2. In a small bowl, whisk together lemon juice, olive oil, salt, and pepper to create the dressing.

3. Drizzle the dressing over the tuna and bean mixture and toss gently to combine.

4. Serve over a bed of mixed greens.

Cooking Time: 10 minutes

6. Veggie and Hummus Wrap

A quick and satisfying lunch option packed with fiber and vitamins.

Ingredients:

- 1 whole wheat tortilla
- 2 tablespoons hummus
- 1/2 cup mixed raw vegetables (e.g., cucumber, bell pepper, carrots)
- 1/4 cup baby spinach leaves
- 1/4 cup sliced avocado
- Salt and pepper to taste

Instructions:

1. Lay the whole wheat tortilla flat.

2. Spread hummus evenly over the tortilla.

3. Add mixed raw vegetables, baby spinach, and sliced avocado.

4. Season with salt and pepper.

5. Roll the tortilla, slice in half, and serve.

Cooking Time: 5 minutes

7. Chickpea and Vegetable Curry

A hearty and flavorful curry with chickpeas and vegetables
to keep you satisfied and nourished.

Ingredients:

- 1 can (15 oz) chickpeas, drained and rinsed
- 1 cup mixed vegetables (e.g., cauliflower, bell pepper, peas)
- 1 onion, finely chopped
- 2 cloves garlic, minced
- 1 tablespoon ginger, minced
- 1 can (14 oz) diced tomatoes
- 1 can (14 oz) coconut milk
- 2 tablespoons curry powder
- Salt and pepper to taste
- Cooked brown rice or quinoa (optional)

Instructions:

1. Heat olive oil in a large skillet or pot over medium heat.

2. Add chopped onion and sauté until translucent.

3. Stir in minced garlic and ginger, and cook for an additional 30 seconds.

4. Add curry powder and cook for 1-2 minutes until fragrant.

5. Add mixed vegetables, chickpeas, diced tomatoes, and coconut milk.

6. Simmer for 15-20 minutes or until vegetables are tender and the sauce thickens.

7. Season with salt and pepper.

8. Serve as is or over cooked brown rice or quinoa.

Cooking Time: 25-30 minutes

8. Turkey and Avocado Salad

A lean protein-packed salad with healthy fats to keep you feeling full and satisfied.

Ingredients:

- 2 cups mixed greens
- 4 oz turkey breast slices
- 1/2 avocado, sliced
- 1/4 cup cherry tomatoes, halved

- 1/4 cup cucumber, sliced

- 2 tablespoons balsamic vinaigrette dressing

- Salt and pepper to taste

Instructions:

1. Arrange mixed greens on a plate.

2. Top with turkey breast slices, sliced avocado, cherry tomatoes, and cucumber.

3. Drizzle balsamic vinaigrette dressing over the salad.

4. Season with salt and pepper.

5. Serve fresh.

Cooking Time: 10 minutes

9. Sweet Potato and Chickpea Salad

A hearty and nutrient-rich salad with sweet potatoes and chickpeas to keep you energized.

Ingredients:

- 2 cups diced sweet potatoes

- 1 can (15 oz) chickpeas, drained and rinsed

- 1/4 cup red onion, finely chopped

- 1/4 cup fresh cilantro, chopped

- Juice of 1 lime
- 2 tablespoons olive oil
- 1 teaspoon ground cumin
- Salt and pepper to taste

Instructions:

1. Preheat the oven to 425°F (220°C).

2. Toss diced sweet potatoes with olive oil, ground cumin, salt, and pepper.

3. Roast in the oven for 20-25 minutes or until tender and slightly crispy.

4. In a large bowl, combine roasted sweet potatoes, chickpeas, red onion, and cilantro.

5. Drizzle lime juice over the salad and toss gently to combine.

6. Serve warm or at room temperature.

Cooking Time: 30-35 minutes

10. Greek Chicken Salad

A Mediterranean-inspired salad with lean protein and vibrant flavors.

Ingredients:

- 2 cups mixed greens
- 4 oz grilled chicken breast, sliced
- 1/4 cup cherry tomatoes, halved
- 1/4 cup cucumber, sliced
- 2 tablespoons Kalamata olives, pitted and sliced
- 2 tablespoons crumbled feta cheese
- 2 tablespoons Greek dressing
- Fresh oregano or basil for garnish (optional)
- Salt and pepper to taste

Instructions:

1. Arrange mixed greens on a plate.

2. Top with grilled chicken breast slices, cherry tomatoes, cucumber, Kalamata olives, and crumbled feta cheese.

3. Drizzle Greek dressing over the salad.

4. Season with salt and pepper.

5. Garnish with fresh oregano or basil if desired.

6. Serve fresh.

Cooking Time: 15 minutes (if chicken is not pre-cooked)

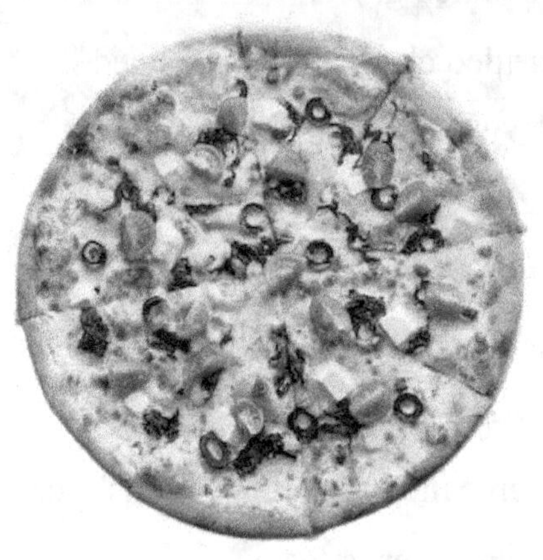

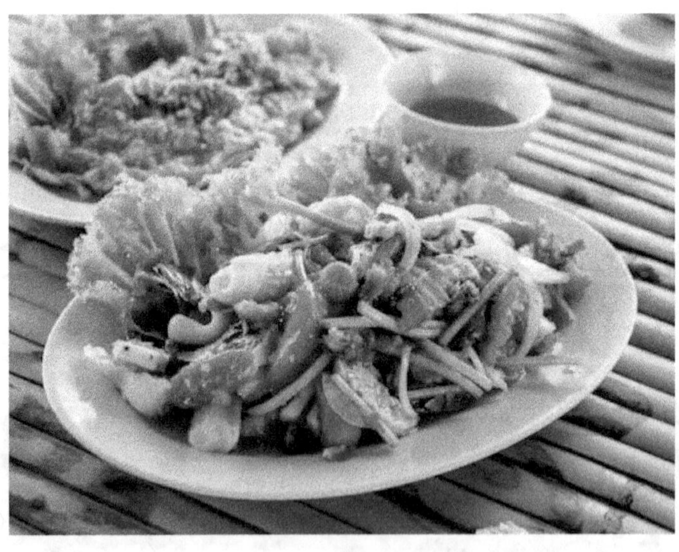

CHAPTER FOUR

Menopause Diet Dinner Recipes

1. Baked Salmon with Lemon and Dill

A simple and flavorful dinner option rich in omega-3 fatty acids and essential nutrients.

Ingredients:

- 4 salmon fillets
- 2 tablespoons olive oil
- 2 tablespoons fresh lemon juice
- 1 tablespoon fresh dill, chopped
- 2 cloves garlic, minced
- Salt and pepper to taste
- Lemon slices for garnish (optional)

Instructions:

1. Preheat the oven to 375°F (190°C).

2. Place salmon fillets on a baking sheet lined with parchment paper.

3. In a small bowl, whisk together olive oil, lemon juice, fresh dill, minced garlic, salt, and pepper.

4. Drizzle the mixture over the salmon fillets.

5. Arrange lemon slices on top.

6. Bake for 15-20 minutes or until the salmon is cooked through and flakes easily with a fork.

7. Serve hot.

Cooking Time: 20-25 minutes

2. Vegetable Stir-Fry with Tofu

A plant-based stir-fry with tofu and colorful vegetables to support overall health during menopause.

Ingredients:

- 1 block (14 oz) extra-firm tofu, cubed
- 2 tablespoons low-sodium soy sauce or tamari
- 1 tablespoon sesame oil
- 1 tablespoon rice vinegar
- 1 teaspoon honey or agave nectar
- 2 cloves garlic, minced
- 1 tablespoon ginger, minced
- 2 cups mixed vegetables (e.g., bell peppers, broccoli, snap peas)

- Cooked brown rice or quinoa for serving (optional)

Instructions:

1. In a bowl, combine cubed tofu, soy sauce, sesame oil, rice vinegar, honey or agave nectar, minced garlic, and minced ginger. Allow the tofu to marinate for 10 minutes.

2. Heat a large skillet or wok over medium-high heat.

3. Add marinated tofu and stir-fry until golden brown on all sides. Remove from the skillet and set aside.

4. In the same skillet, add mixed vegetables and stir-fry until tender-crisp.

5. Return tofu to the skillet and toss to combine.

6. Serve over cooked brown rice or quinoa if desired.

Cooking Time: 20 minutes

3. Stuffed Bell Peppers

A wholesome dinner option that combines lean ground turkey and a variety of vegetables.

Ingredients:

- 4 bell peppers, any color
- 1/2 lb lean ground turkey
- 1 cup cooked brown rice
- 1 cup diced tomatoes (canned or fresh)
- 1/2 cup black beans (canned, drained, and rinsed)
- 1/2 cup corn kernels (fresh or frozen)
- 1/2 teaspoon chili powder
- 1/2 teaspoon cumin
- Salt and pepper to taste
- Shredded cheese for topping (optional)

Instructions:

1. Preheat the oven to 375°F (190°C).

2. Cut the tops off the bell peppers and remove seeds and membranes.

3. In a skillet, cook ground turkey until browned and cooked through.

4. In a large bowl, combine cooked ground turkey, cooked brown rice, diced tomatoes, black beans, corn, chili powder, cumin, salt, and pepper.

5. Stuff each bell pepper with the turkey and rice mixture.

6. Place stuffed peppers in a baking dish and cover with aluminum foil.

7. Bake for 25-30 minutes or until peppers are tender.

8. If desired, remove the foil, sprinkle with shredded cheese, and bake for an additional 5 minutes or until cheese is melted and bubbly.

9. Serve hot.

Cooking Time: 35-40 minutes

4. Mediterranean Chickpea Salad

A refreshing and nutritious salad with chickpeas, vegetables, and Mediterranean flavors.

Ingredients:

- 2 cans (15 oz each) chickpeas, drained and rinsed
- 1 cup cherry tomatoes, halved
- 1 cucumber, diced
- 1/2 red onion, finely chopped
- 1/4 cup Kalamata olives, pitted and sliced

- 1/4 cup fresh parsley, chopped
- Juice of 1 lemon
- 2 tablespoons extra-virgin olive oil
- 1 teaspoon dried oregano
- Salt and pepper to taste
- Feta cheese for garnish (optional)

Instructions:

1. In a large bowl, combine chickpeas, cherry tomatoes, cucumber, red onion, Kalamata olives, and fresh parsley.

2. In a small bowl, whisk together lemon juice, extra-virgin olive oil, dried oregano, salt, and pepper to create the dressing.

3. Drizzle the dressing over the salad and toss gently to combine.

4. If desired, garnish with crumbled feta cheese before serving.

5. Serve chilled.

Cooking Time: 15 minutes

5. Baked Chicken Thighs with Roasted Vegetables

A wholesome dinner featuring baked chicken thighs and a medley of roasted vegetables.

Ingredients:

- 4 bone-in, skinless chicken thighs
- 2 cups mixed vegetables (e.g., carrots, Brussels sprouts, and potatoes)
- 2 tablespoons olive oil
- 2 cloves garlic, minced
- 1 teaspoon dried rosemary
- Salt and pepper to taste

Instructions:

1. Preheat the oven to 400°F (200°C).

2. In a large bowl, toss mixed vegetables with olive oil, minced garlic, dried rosemary, salt, and pepper.

3. Place chicken thighs on a baking sheet.

4. Arrange seasoned vegetables around the chicken.

5. Bake for 30-35 minutes or until the chicken is cooked through and the vegetables are tender.

6. Serve hot.

Cooking Time: 35-40 minutes

6. Shrimp and Broccoli Stir-Fry

A quick and flavorful stir-fry that combines shrimp and broccoli for a protein-packed dinner.

Ingredients:

- 1 lb large shrimp, peeled and deveined
- 2 cups broccoli florets
- 1 red bell pepper, sliced
- 1/4 cup low-sodium soy sauce or tamari
- 2 tablespoons hoisin sauce
- 1 tablespoon honey or agave nectar
- 2 cloves garlic, minced
- 1 tablespoon ginger, minced
- 1 teaspoon cornstarch
- Cooked brown rice for serving

Instructions:

1. In a bowl, whisk together soy sauce, hoisin sauce, honey or agave nectar, minced garlic, minced ginger, and cornstarch to create the sauce.

2. Heat a large skillet or wok over high heat.

3. Add shrimp and stir-fry for 2-3 minutes or until pink and cooked through. Remove from the skillet and set aside.

4. In the same skillet, add broccoli florets and red bell pepper slices. Stir-fry for 3-4 minutes or until tender-crisp.

5. Return cooked shrimp to the skillet and pour the sauce over the shrimp and vegetables.

6. Cook for an additional 2-3 minutes or until the sauce thickens.

7. Serve over cooked brown rice.

Cooking Time: 20 minutes

7. Spinach and Mushroom Stuffed Chicken Breast

A savory dinner option featuring stuffed chicken breast with spinach and mushrooms.

Ingredients:

- 4 boneless, skinless chicken breasts
- 2 cups fresh spinach leaves
- 1 cup sliced mushrooms
- 1/4 cup low-fat cream cheese
- 2 cloves garlic, minced
- 1/2 teaspoon dried thyme
- Salt and pepper to taste
- Olive oil for cooking

Instructions:

1. Preheat the oven to 375°F (190°C).

2. Cut a pocket into each chicken breast.

3. In a skillet, heat olive oil over medium heat.

4. Add sliced mushrooms and sauté until tender.

5. Add minced garlic and cook for an additional 30 seconds.

6. Stir in fresh spinach leaves and cook until wilted.

7. Remove the skillet from heat and stir in low-fat cream cheese, dried thyme, salt, and pepper.

8. Stuff each chicken breast with the spinach and mushroom mixture.

9. Place stuffed chicken breasts on a baking sheet lined with parchment paper.

10. Bake for 25-30 minutes or until the chicken is cooked through and no longer pink.

11. Serve hot.

Cooking Time: 30-35 minutes

8. Lentil and Vegetable Soup

A hearty and nutritious soup with lentils and a variety of vegetables.

Ingredients:

- 1 cup dried green or brown lentils, rinsed and drained
- 1 onion, finely chopped
- 2 carrots, diced
- 2 celery stalks, diced
- 2 cloves garlic, minced
- 1 can (14 oz) diced tomatoes
- 6 cups vegetable broth
- 1 teaspoon dried thyme
- 1 teaspoon dried rosemary

- Salt and pepper to taste

- Fresh parsley for garnish (optional)

Instructions:

1. In a large pot, heat olive oil over medium heat.

2. Add chopped onion, diced carrots, and diced celery. Sauté until vegetables are softened.

3. Stir in minced garlic and cook for an additional 30 seconds.

4. Add dried lentils, diced tomatoes, vegetable broth, dried thyme, dried rosemary, salt, and pepper.

5. Bring to a boil, then reduce heat to low and simmer for 25-30 minutes or until lentils are tender.

6. Garnish with fresh parsley before serving.

7. Serve hot.

Cooking Time: 35-40 minutes

9. Teriyaki Tofu and Broccoli

A flavorful and plant-based dinner option featuring teriyaki tofu and crisp broccoli.

Ingredients:

- 1 block (14 oz) extra-firm tofu, cubed
- 2 cups broccoli florets
- 1/4 cup low-sodium teriyaki sauce
- 2 tablespoons sesame seeds
- 2 green onions, sliced (for garnish)
- Cooked brown rice for serving

Instructions:

1. In a bowl, toss cubed tofu with teriyaki sauce and sesame seeds. Allow tofu to marinate for 10 minutes.

2. Heat a large skillet or wok over medium-high heat.

3. Add marinated tofu and stir-fry until golden brown on all sides. Remove from the skillet and set aside.

4. In the same skillet, add broccoli florets and stir-fry for 3-4 minutes or until tender-crisp.

5. Return cooked tofu to the skillet and toss to combine.

6. Serve over cooked brown rice, garnished with sliced green onions.

Cooking Time: 20 minutes

10. Butternut Squash and Kale Pasta

A comforting and nutrient-rich pasta dish with roasted butternut squash and sautéed kale.

Ingredients:

- 8 oz whole wheat pasta
- 2 cups diced butternut squash
- 2 cups kale leaves, stemmed and chopped
- 2 cloves garlic, minced
- 2 tablespoons olive oil
- 1/4 cup grated Parmesan cheese
- Salt and pepper to taste

Instructions:

1. Preheat the oven to 400°F (200°C).

2. Toss diced butternut squash with 1 tablespoon of olive oil,

salt, and pepper. Roast for 20-25 minutes or until tender and slightly caramelized.

3. Cook pasta according to package instructions until al dente. Drain and set aside.

4. In a large skillet, heat 1 tablespoon of olive oil over medium heat.

5. Add minced garlic and sauté for 30 seconds.

6. Stir in chopped kale and sauté until wilted.

7. Combine cooked pasta, roasted butternut squash, sautéed kale, and grated Parmesan cheese in a large bowl.

8. Toss to combine and season with additional salt and pepper if needed.

9. Serve hot.

Cooking Time: 35-40 minutes (including roasting the butternut squash)

Menopause Diet Snacks Recipes

1. Greek Yogurt and Berry Parfait

A satisfying and nutritious snack loaded with protein, probiotics, and antioxidants.

Ingredients:

- 1 cup Greek yogurt
- 1/2 cup mixed berries (e.g., blueberries, strawberries, raspberries)
- 1 tablespoon honey or agave nectar
- 1/4 cup granola

Instructions:

1. In a glass or bowl, layer Greek yogurt.

2. Add a layer of mixed berries on top of the yogurt.

3. Drizzle honey or agave nectar over the berries.

4. Sprinkle granola on top.

5. Serve immediately.

Preparation Time: 5 minutes

2. Sliced Apple with Almond Butter

A simple and satisfying snack that combines the natural sweetness of apples with the creaminess of almond butter.

Ingredients:

- 1 apple, sliced
- 2 tablespoons almond butter
- Cinnamon for sprinkling (optional)

Instructions:

1. Slice the apple into thin wedges.

2. Dip each apple slice into almond butter.

3. Sprinkle with cinnamon if desired.

4. Enjoy!

Preparation Time: 5 minutes

3. Veggie Sticks with Hummus

A crunchy and nutrient-rich snack that pairs fresh vegetable sticks with creamy hummus.

Ingredients:

- Assorted vegetable sticks (e.g., carrots, celery, cucumber, bell peppers)
- 1/4 cup hummus

Instructions:

1. Wash and cut the vegetables into sticks.

2. Serve with hummus for dipping.

3. Enjoy the crunch and flavor!

Preparation Time: 10 minutes

4. Avocado and Tomato Salsa

A zesty and heart-healthy snack featuring creamy avocado and flavorful tomato salsa.

Ingredients:

- 1 ripe avocado, diced
- 1/2 cup diced tomatoes
- 1/4 cup red onion, finely chopped
- 1/4 cup fresh cilantro, chopped
- Juice of 1 lime

- Salt and pepper to taste

- Baked whole-grain tortilla chips for dipping

Instructions:

1. In a bowl, combine diced avocado, diced tomatoes, chopped red onion, and chopped cilantro.

2. Squeeze lime juice over the mixture and season with salt and pepper.

3. Serve with whole-grain tortilla chips for dipping.

4. Enjoy this tasty and nutrient-rich snack!

Preparation Time: 10 minutes

5. Trail Mix

A convenient and energy-boosting snack combining a variety of nuts, seeds, and dried fruits.

Ingredients:

- 1/4 cup almonds

- 1/4 cup walnuts

- 1/4 cup pumpkin seeds

- 1/4 cup dried cranberries

- 1/4 cup dark chocolate chips (optional)

Instructions:

1. Mix all the ingredients together in a bowl.

2. Portion into snack-sized bags for convenient on-the-go munching.

3. Enjoy this balanced and satisfying snack.

Preparation Time: 5 minutes

6. Cottage Cheese with Pineapple

A protein-rich snack that combines creamy cottage cheese with sweet and tangy pineapple.

Ingredients:

- 1/2 cup low-fat cottage cheese
- 1/2 cup fresh pineapple chunks (or canned pineapple in juice, drained)

Instructions:

1. Spoon cottage cheese into a bowl.

2. Top with fresh pineapple chunks.

3. Enjoy this quick and filling snack.

Preparation Time: 5 minutes

7. Almond and Date Energy Balls

Homemade energy balls that are easy to make and provide a boost of sustained energy.

Ingredients:

- 1 cup pitted dates
- 1/2 cup almonds
- 1/4 cup unsweetened cocoa powder
- 1 tablespoon honey or maple syrup
- 1/2 teaspoon vanilla extract
- Pinch of salt
- Shredded coconut for rolling (optional)

Instructions:

1. In a food processor, combine dates, almonds, cocoa powder, honey or maple syrup, vanilla extract, and a pinch of salt.

2. Process until the mixture forms a sticky dough.

3. Roll the dough into small balls.

4. If desired, roll the balls in shredded coconut.

5. Refrigerate for at least 30 minutes before enjoying.

Preparation Time: 20 minutes (including chilling)

8. Edamame with Sea Salt

A protein-packed snack that combines steamed edamame with a sprinkle of sea salt.

Ingredients:

- 1 cup frozen edamame in pods
- Sea salt for sprinkling

Instructions:

1. Cook edamame according to package instructions, typically by boiling or steaming for a few minutes.

2. Drain and let cool slightly.

3. Sprinkle with sea salt.

4. Pop the edamame pods open and enjoy the tender, salty beans inside.

Preparation Time: 10 minutes

9. Cucumber and Tzatziki

A refreshing and hydrating snack featuring cucumber slices paired with creamy tzatziki sauce.

Ingredients:

- 1 cucumber, sliced
- 1/4 cup tzatziki sauce

Instructions:

1. Slice the cucumber into thin rounds.

2. Serve with tzatziki sauce for dipping.

3. Enjoy the cool and crisp flavors!

Preparation Time: 5 minutes

10. Rice Cake with Peanut Butter and Banana

A satisfying snack that combines the crunch of rice cakes with the creaminess of peanut butter and the sweetness of bananas.

Ingredients:

- 1 rice cake
- 1 tablespoon peanut butter (or almond butter)
- 1/2 banana, thinly sliced
- Honey for drizzling (optional)

Instructions:

1. Spread peanut butter onto the rice cake.

2. Top with banana slices.

3. If desired, drizzle honey over the top for added sweetness.

4. Enjoy this quick and delightful snack!

Preparation Time: 5 minutes

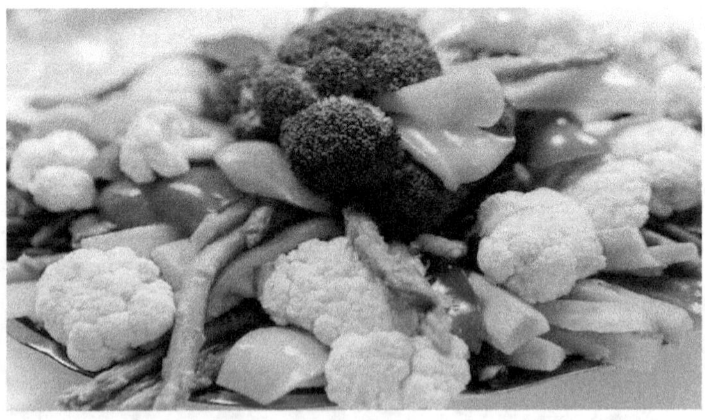

CONCLUSION

The menopause diet plays a vital role in helping women navigate the physical and hormonal changes that occur during this transformative phase of life. As women transition through menopause, their nutritional needs shift, and making the right dietary choices can significantly impact their overall well-being and quality of life.

The menopause diet is all about balance and moderation. It emphasizes whole, nutrient-rich foods while limiting processed and sugary items. By incorporating a variety of foods such as fruits, vegetables, lean proteins, whole grains, and healthy fats, women can better manage common menopausal symptoms like weight gain, hot flashes, mood swings, and bone density loss. A key focus of the menopause diet is ensuring an adequate intake of essential nutrients. Calcium and vitamin D are crucial for bone health, as the risk of osteoporosis increases post-menopause. Incorporating dairy products, leafy greens, fortified foods, and supplements if necessary can help maintain strong bones. Omega-3 fatty acids, found in fatty fish, flaxseeds, and walnuts, can alleviate inflammation and promote heart health.

Fiber-rich foods like whole grains, legumes, and vegetables can help manage weight and control blood sugar levels, which can become more challenging during menopause. Moreover, phytoestrogen-rich foods, such as soy products and flaxseeds, can potentially mitigate hormonal fluctuations and reduce the severity of hot flashes. Hydration is also crucial, as menopausal women may experience increased susceptibility to dehydration. Drinking an adequate amount of water and consuming hydrating foods like watermelon, cucumbers, and citrus fruits can help maintain optimal fluid balance. Overall, the menopause diet is not just about managing symptoms; it's about empowering women to embrace this life stage with vitality and resilience. A well-rounded diet, combined with a healthy lifestyle, can support women as they transition through menopause, enabling them to enjoy a fulfilling and active life beyond this transformative period. It's important for women to consult with healthcare professionals or registered dietitians to tailor their diet plans to their specific needs and ensure they receive the necessary guidance for a smooth and healthy menopausal journey.